The Depression Cure

*The 11-Step Program To Naturally Beat
Depression For Life*

Table of Contents

Introduction

Depression is one of the most widespread mental disorders in the world - an estimated 400 million people suffer from the condition and over 50% of all people who commit suicide are affected by it. These statistics are extremely alarming, especially when considering that suicide takes more lives than war, murder and natural disasters combined.

Major depressive disorder, the most severe form of depression, is classified as a serious mental illness that requires medical attention and treatment. Over the years, antidepressants have been the most commonly prescribed treatment for depression, and the general opinion is that they are safe and effective.

However, in recent times, antidepressants have raised a multitude of concerns due to their wide range of side effects which include suicide, sleep disturbances, weight gain, increased relapse rates and loss of sexual desire, just to name a few. Many patients who have taken antidepressants have had their depression worsen over the long-term through a process called antidepressant-induced chronic depression. The FDA has even instructed all antidepressant drug manufacturers to add a black warning label (the most serious one) to their medication.

A recent article published in the journal *Frontiers in Psychology* says, "The weight of current evidence suggests that, in general, antidepressants are neither safe nor effective; they appear to do more harm than good."

Dr Mark Hyman, eight-time #1 New York Times bestselling author, openly says in an article published on the Huffington Post, "Antidepressants don't work... the pharmaceutical industry and Food and Drug Administration (FDA) have deliberately deceived us into believing that they DO work. As a physician, this is frightening to me."

The purpose of this book is not to make a case against antidepressants. Medication can certainly be valuable in some cases. However, the widespread belief that antidepressants are the best solution for treating depression is ill-founded, sometimes fatal and must be challenged.

The aim of this book is to provide alternatives solutions for overcoming depression without having to resort to prescription drugs and endure their side effects.

Depression is beatable – and the 11 steps outlined in this book will show exactly how you can naturally overcome it while improving your overall health and happiness. .

Step 1 - Understanding Depression

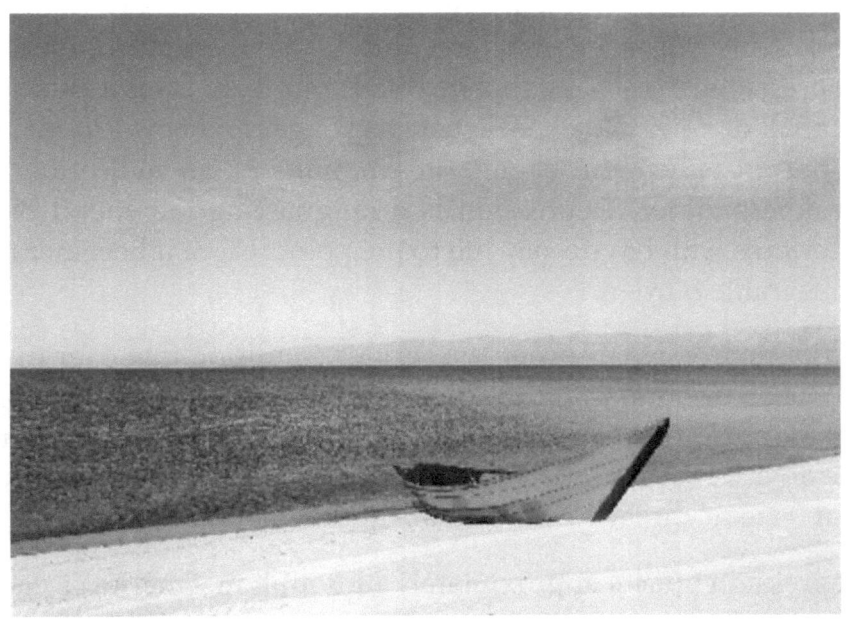

"A problem clearly stated is a problem half solved."
Dorothea Brande

There is a great deal of confusion around the idea of depression. The term "depressed" or "depression" has been used to describe everything from the state of the economy (such as the 1929 Great Depression) to how people feel after a break-up or an exhausting day at the office.

In everyday conversation, the term is associated with temporary feelings of sadness or dejection, but the truth is that depression is much more profound than that. We all experience feeling sad, dejected or blasé from time to time. Those feelings are normal and simply part of the vicissitudes of life.

However, in a clinical context, the word depression is entirely different. It doesn't merely denote a brief spell of sadness or feeling down in the dumps. Depression is first and foremost a crippling form of mental illness – its precise label is *major depressive disorder*, but we call it depression for short. Depression isn't what happens when your team loses a game of football or when a pickpocket steals your brand new IPhone. It is not an ephemeral change in emotions or an indication of weakness either. Depression is a long lasting low mood that interferes with day-to-day life to the point where it becomes an unbearable burden.

Major depressive disorder is a serious condition that over time damages the brain and the body. Unfortunately many people still confuse this condition with mere feelings of sadness and the advice that we hear so often ("suck it up" or "just snap out of it") stems directly from this misunderstanding.

Depression affects approximately 14.8 million Americans each year, and the average age for the symptoms to manifest is around 32 years. This roughly translates to about 1 in 10 Americans suffering from varying levels of the illness, and this number is projected to increase by up to 20% in the coming years.

People who suffer from depression often find themselves paralyzed by it. They no longer take pleasure in the hobbies and relationships that they once enjoyed and find it difficult to function normally in daily life. Depression often feels like a quiet despair, a downward spiral with no light at the end of the tunnel where you can easily end up questioning your entire purpose in life.

What Causes Depression

Depression is often a reaction to devastating life changes such as the death of a loved one or a painful divorce, but the following factors can be catalysts as well:

- **Psychiatric illnesses**: A major depressive disorder often works in combination with other mental illnesses such as anxiety, borderline personality disorder, schizophrenia, and bipolar disorder.

- **Non-psychiatric illnesses**: Patients who struggle with diseases like cancer, diabetes, or Addison's disease sometimes grapple with depression as a result. A nutritional deficiency can also cause a rather low mood.

- **Medical treatments or drugs**: Certain prescribed medications can lead to depressive symptoms. The use of sleeping pills is correlated to the rise of such symptoms. Prescription drugs for ailments such as high blood pressure are also likely causes.

- **Hepatitis C**: Patients who undergo interferon therapy are at risk of developing major depressive disorder.

- **The weather**: Lack of sunlight exposure can cause you to feel a little gray over an extended period of time. This is why some people struggle with depressive symptoms during the winter when the daylight supply is insufficient.

- **Substance abuse**: Individuals who consume drugs, alcohol, and/or nicotine are at higher risk of developing major depressive disorder.

- **Diet**: Certain foods can exacerbate depressive symptoms. This will be discussed further in the *Nutrition* section of this book.

Symptoms of Depression

In order to find out if you or a loved one is suffering from major depressive disorder, here are specific symptoms to look out for:

- **Extreme changes in appetite:** Suddenly feeling ravenous or exhibiting very little appetite are both possible symptoms of major depressive disorder.

- **Excessive weight loss or gain**: In line with the previous symptom, individuals suffering from depression tend to either gain or lose weight in a short period of time.

- **Abnormal sleeping patterns**: These include insomnia, waking up during the night for no apparent reason, or even hypersomnia (oversleeping).

- **Lack of interest**: Depressed people often feel as though they no longer enjoy the everyday activities that used to bring them so much joy and happiness.

- **Lower libido**: The desire to engage in intimate relations is considerably lessened.

- **Loss of energy**: Feeling exhausted and drained all the time. Even small tasks such as placing clothes in the hamper or even getting out of bed may seem extremely demanding.

- **Inability to concentrate**: Difficulty in remembering things or focusing can also be a symptom of depression.

- **Broken self-esteem**: Depression is often accompanied by pronounced feelings of worthlessness that can destroy one's self-esteem.

- **Aches and pains:** Major depressive disorder can cause increased occurrences of headaches, stomach pain, and back pain.

- **Increased agitation or irritability:** Constantly feeling on edge and becoming short-tempered are also symptoms.

These symptoms may seem overwhelming, and if you happen to be experiencing them, don't worry. Depression is beatable, and the next few steps will show you exactly how to overcome this condition without using any prescription drugs.

Step 2 - Restoring Your Self-Esteem

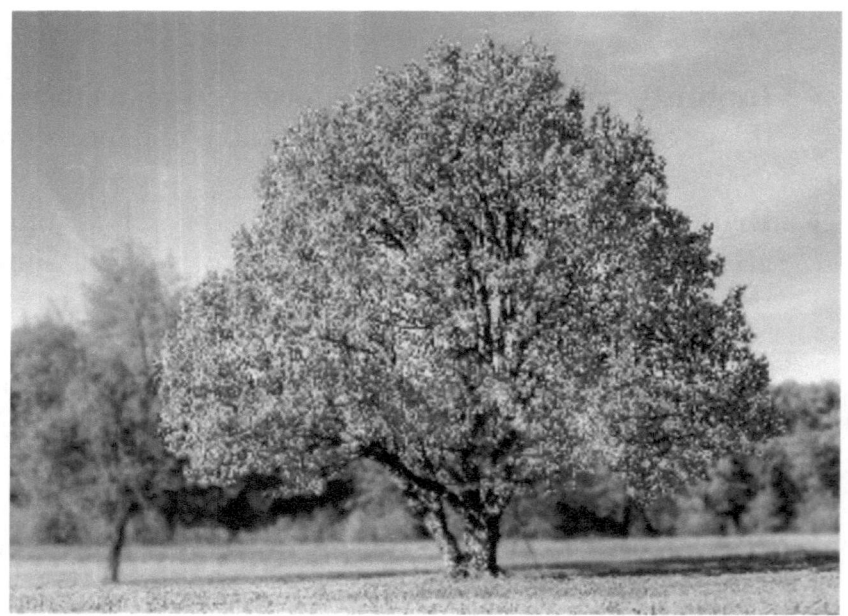

"You're imperfect, and you're wired for struggle, but you are worthy of love and belonging."
Brene Brown

Depression often comes with feelings of worthlessness and inadequacy that can be very harmful to anyone on the path to recovery. In order to beat depression, these feelings must be challenged and replaced with more positive, empowering ones. Restoring your self-esteem is a critical part of the recovery process. As Dr Louis Hart eloquently says, "Self esteem is as important to our well-being as legs are to a table. It is essential for physical and mental health and for happiness"

Self-esteem is the voice deep inside you that tells you whether you are good enough. It is your belief about your own worth and value in the world. Self-esteem is the invisible force that dictates every choice and decision you make – it affects virtually every area of your life – your relationships, health, level of happiness and even your finances.

Best-selling author Iyanla Vanzant puts it beautifully: "Everything that happens to you is a reflection of what you believe about yourself. We cannot outperform our level of self-esteem. We cannot draw to ourselves more than we think we are worth." The truth is, people don't get what they deserve out of life, they get what they deeply believe they deserve. This is why cultivating your self-esteem is so important if you want to overcome depression and live a happy, fulfilling life.

Here are some signs of low self-esteem that you may be able to recognize in yourself or a loved one:

- Having a hard time accepting compliments

- Being overly concerned with how other people perceive you

- Being highly sensitive to criticism

- Comparing yourself to everyone you encounter

- Avoiding conflict at all costs

- Apologizing too often

- Putting other people down

If you do recognize some of these signs in yourself, don't worry. The good news is you are in complete control of your level of self-esteem. All you have to do is challenge the negative beliefs that you hold about yourself. Here are some practical steps to achieve higher self-esteem:

Acknowledge your positive qualities

Make a list of three things that you like about yourself every evening before you go to bed. You can keep your lists in a "self-esteem" journal that you can refer to when you are in need of a positive boost.

Take control of your self-talk

Become aware of the negative things you say to yourself on a daily basis. The way you consistently talk to yourself has a massive impact on your self-esteem. Replace your inner critic with positive, self-compassionate self-talk.

Surround yourself with positive people

You are the average of the 5 people you hang around the most with. Avoid people who bring you down and go out of your comfort zone to be around positive people who make you feel better about yourself.

View mistakes as opportunities to learn

Einstein says, "Anyone who has never made a mistake has never tried anything new" Don't dwell on your mistakes, simply learn from them, use them to improve and move on.

Set yourself a challenge

Set a goal that is within your reach, but not too easy, and go out and achieve it. Accomplishing goals can significantly boost your self-esteem and potentially propel you into a positive spiral of success.

Realize that good enough is perfect

Don't get held back by the desire to be perfect. Perfectionism is often merely an excuse for not taking action. Strive for effort rather than perfection.

To improve your self-esteem, the only thing you need to internalize is that there is no reason why you're not enough. Let the truth of that statement sink in for a second and realize that this cannot be disputed.

Every human being on this planet is worthy of love and belonging. We were all born mentally healthy. Babies do not ever get depressed - they live in a continual state of mental well-being because well-being is our true nature. Babies do not ever need to struggle for worthiness because worthiness is our true nature.

Once you recognize that your default, natural state is one of peace, love and happiness, you begin to awaken and you realize what Michael Neil says in *The Inside Out Revolution:* "There's nothing you need to do, be, have, get, change, practice, or learn in order to be happy, loving, and whole."

Step 3 - Nutrition

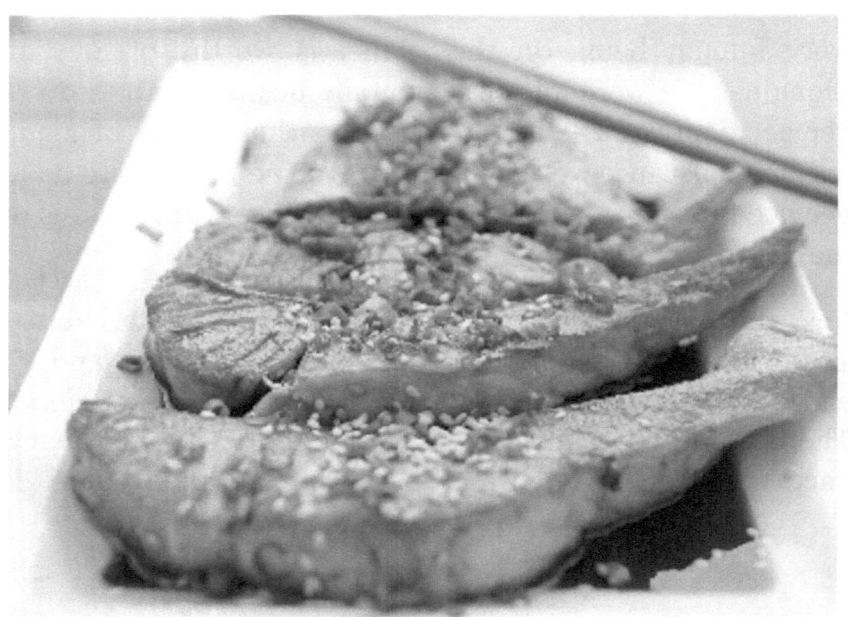

"The only way to keep your health is to eat what you don't want, drink what you don't like, and do what you'd rather not."
Mark Twain

The wellbeing of the mind is intrinsically linked to that of the body's. A healthy body equals a healthy mind, as the former provides nourishment and energy to the latter. To improve your mental health and combat depression, here are 4 super foods to incorporate into your diet:

- **Salmon**: The pink fish is rich in omega-3 fatty acids, an essential substance that fights free radicals and keeps your brain sharp. A Norwegian study of around 22,000 participants has shown that people who regularly take omega-3 fatty acids are about 30% less likely to suffer from depression. Omega-3 fatty acids improve your blood circulation, relieve inflammation and as a result reduce depressive episodes triggered by brain inflammation. Salmon can also be substituted with other oily fish such as mackerel, tuna, bluefish, or even with dietary supplements.

- **Walnuts**: Walnuts are a great plant-based alternative if you aren't keen on eating fish but still want to get the precious omega-3 fatty acids. Consuming walnuts will improve your mental health and alleviate your depressive symptoms.

- **Dark green, leafy vegetables**: The green color of these vegetables is an indication of their high vitamin B6 content. Vitamin B6 is another nutrient that is essential for your brain's health. Go for the darker-hued romaine lettuce over the pale iceberg ones, or load up on spinach and broccoli. If you aren't too keen on your greens, you can always mix them into a smoothie with fruits that you love (bananas, pineapples, oranges...)

- **Green tea**: Green tea is packed full of antioxidants that protect your cells from damage by environmental and dietary toxins. Several studies have found low levels of antioxidants to be correlated with symptoms of depression. Besides, tea contains high levels of theanine, a naturally occurring amino acid, which is effective for relieving stress and relaxing the mind.

In addition to incorporating these healthy foods into your diet, it is just as important to minimize your intake of the following:

- **Processed foods**: They contain high amounts of sodium and refined sugar, two things that cause your blood pressure to spike and your body to feel sluggish.

- **Coffee or carbonated beverages**: The high caffeine content of these drinks will exacerbate your depressive/anxious symptoms, since they cause your pulse to increase. Excessive consumption of such can lead to feelings of increased agitation.

- **Alcohol**: If you are depressed, alcohol is one of the worst things you could put into your body. It is classified as a central nervous system depressant so it will only aggravate your condition.

Finally, make sure to drink plenty of water in order to keep yourself hydrated. Sufficient water intake will flush out toxins and impurities from your body, improve your circulation, reduce inflammation and thus alleviate your symptoms.

Step 4 – Exercise

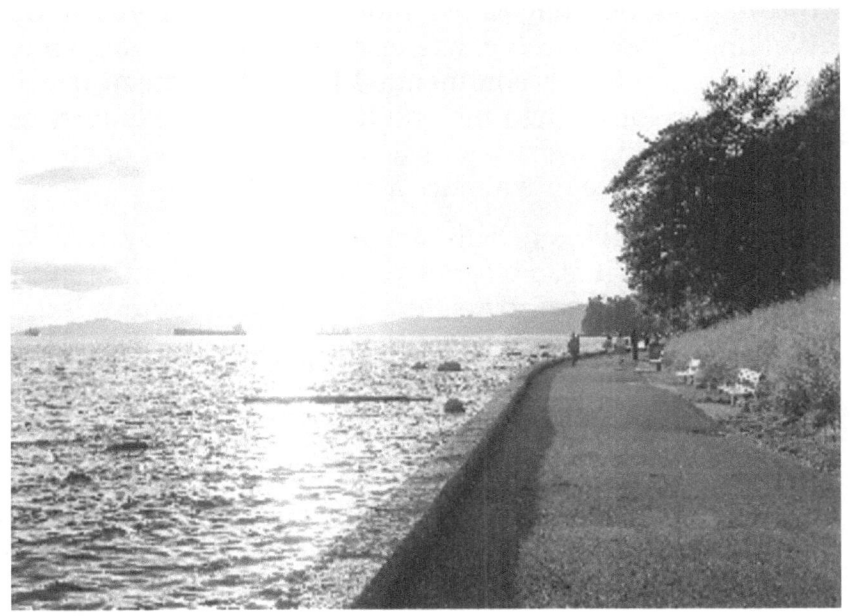

"To enjoy the glow of good health, you must exercise."
Gene Tunney

Exercise is proven to significantly reduce symptoms of depression. Several studies have shown that people who exercise regularly benefit from a positive boost in mood and much lower rates of depression.

When you exercise, your brain releases feel-good chemicals called endorphins. Theses endorphins produce a positive feeling in your body, similar to the effect of morphine. Exercise also provides a healthy outlet for relieving stress and frustration and over time exercise causes your brain to rewire itself in positive ways. Being engaged in physical activity also keeps your mind too busy to dwell on the feelings of guilt and worthlessness that often accompany depression.

Here are ways to incorporate exercise into your daily routine to help you fight off the blues:

- **Take a walk**: Studies have shown that walking as little as fifteen minutes a day can significantly improve your mood. Walking is an aerobic exercise that lowers your blood pressure and it is recommended if you have been battling depression for a long time and have become sedentary as a result. Walking everyday at a leisurely pace is one of the best ways to ease into a more active lifestyle.

- **Try a yoga class**: This ancient art not only develops flexibility, but it also teaches you breathing techniques that will help you relieve stress, tension and relax your mind.

- **Jump on a trampoline or use a skipping rope**: The bouncing motion will make you feel more upbeat and the physical exertion will get your endorphins flowing.

- **Attend a tai chi class**: The gentle and flowing movements in tai chi are great for centering your mind and for relieving frazzled nerves. The fact that most tai chi classes are conducted in groups also helps - the relatively social atmosphere will banish feelings of isolation and loneliness.

- **Break into a run**: The combined cardiovascular and aerobic exercise that running provides will boost your spirits and drastically improve your mood. The sustained physical activity involved in running stimulates the production of endorphins, which will naturally make you feel happier.

When it comes to exercise as a treatment for depression, it is important to remember that a little commitment goes a long way. Start small, maybe with a short walk outside in the morning, and build your way up gradually. If you can overcome the inclination to remain inactive and get yourself to move your body, you will be well on your way to beating depression.

Step 5 - Mindfulness Meditation

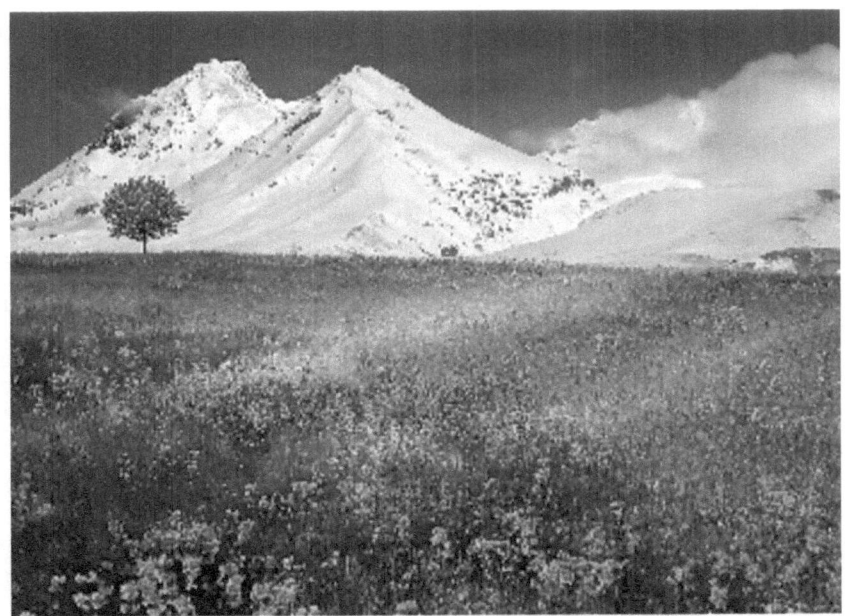

"In meditation, I can let go of everything. I'm not Hugh Jackman. I'm not a dad. I'm not a husband. I'm just dipping into that powerful source that creates everything..."
Hugh Jackman

A study conducted by psychologists at the University of Exeter in the UK has shown mindfulness meditation to be more effective than drugs or even counseling for fighting depression in the long run. In the study, a number of participants were instructed to practice mindfulness meditation 30 minutes a day for 8 weeks. Fifteen months after the training, only 47% of people who suffered from long-term depression relapsed, compared to 60% of those who used anti-depressant drugs without doing meditation.

Meditation changes the structure of your brain through a process called neuroplasticity. Theses positive changes in brain structure explain why regular meditators report a myriad of improvements in their lives. Mindfulness meditation is one of the most popular types of meditation and it involves being fully aware and conscious of the present moment. It is an inner journey that takes you beyond the mind, into a place of stillness where you experience peace, joy and happiness. To practice mindfulness meditation, simply follow these steps:

- **Start small**: There is no "right" amount of time to meditate for. If you're a beginner, don't fall into the trap of trying to meditate for hours on end. Your mind simply isn't trained to sustain it. You can start with as little as 5 minutes of daily meditation and gradually build your way up from there.

- **Get comfortable and fix your posture**: Wear comfortable clothes that will not distract or restrict you. Your posture is important. Your back should be relaxed and upright. You can sit on a chair with your hands on your lap, or on the floor on top of a cushion with your legs crossed.

- **Focus on your breath**: Purposefully direct your attention to the changing sensations of your breath. Become aware of the air flowing in and out of your nostrils. Notice how each breath is slightly different. Be aware of the subtle gap between your incoming and outcoming breath. When thoughts pop up in your mind, observe them without identifying with them; accept them as they are and gently return your attention to your breathing. Repeat this process during your entire meditation.

When you practice meditation, you gain control over your mind, you break the cycle of seeking stimulation from the external world and you learn to draw your state from within. Meditation is truly a transformative experience that can have profound effects not just on your mind, but on virtually every aspect of your life – your body, relationships, health and even your career. If you want to find out more about meditation, I invite you to check out *The Meditation Beginner's Bible* (http://amzn.to/1MR7wlu). This book will show you how to instill simple meditation techniques into your daily routine, inevitably leading you to a more peaceful, happier and healthier life.

Step 6 - Morning Routine

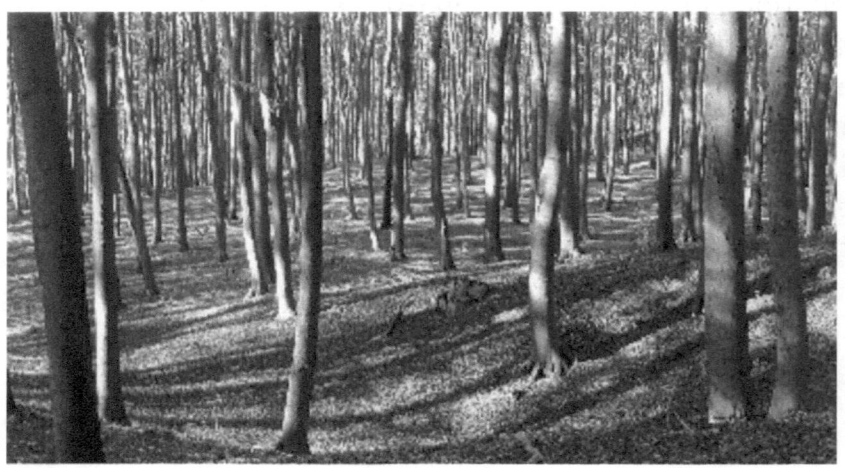

"Morning is an important time of day, because how you spend your morning can often tell you what kind of day you are going to have."
Lemony Snicket

One common complaint amongst people who suffer from depression is that they sometimes cannot distinguish one day from the next. They often feel as though they are stuck in a never-ending cycle of monotonous existence with no real purpose. One day seems to just melt into the next, and life appears pointless.

Depression can make you feel unenthusiastic about getting out of bed and getting on with life, as negative thoughts often hit you as soon as you wake. This is why developing a morning routine that you look forward to is important as it adds structure to your life and helps you to begin each day on a the right foot.

A powerful morning routine will empower you to be at your best everyday, it will set the tone for the rest of your day and is without a doubt one of the most powerful habits you can add to your life. Here are 7 steps for creating a game-changing morning routine:

Smile

In one study, patients who were diagnosed with depression were instructed to look in the mirror and smile at themselves for 20 minutes every day. After four weeks of doing this, not one of them was still depressed. Smiling changes your biochemistry and immediately puts you in a more positive state.

Breathe

Oxygen is the most important thing that your body requires. By breathing deeply into your stomach for a few seconds every morning, you actively cleanse and revitalize the cells of your body.

Drink Water

After oxygen, water is the next most important element that your body needs – your body weight is 70% water and you are the most dehydrated right after you wake up. This is why it's so important to drink water as part of your morning routine.

Feed Your Mind

Read a passage from an inspirational book. If you are religious, you can read a page or two from the book of your faith. Feeding your mind with positive thoughts first thing in the morning will have tremendous impact on the rest of your day.

Stretch

Elongating your limbs and straightening your spine will realign your posture and make you feel better. Stretching can also work out kinks in your back and neck and release some tension.

Make a green smoothie

Adding a green smoothie to your breakfast is one of the healthiest ways to start your day. Green smoothies are easy to digest and offer pure nutrition to your body. All you have to do is mix your favorite fruits with any green, leafy vegetables such as kale, spinach, and lettuce.

Step 7 - Social Contact

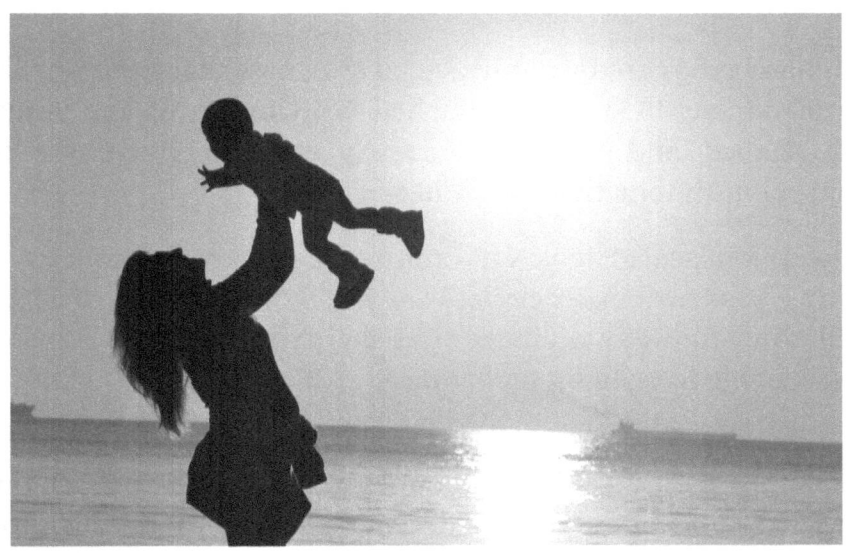

"Man is by nature a social animal; an individual who is unsocial naturally and not accidentally is either beneath our notice or more than human."
Aristotle

Research has found low levels of social contact to be associated with depression and other forms on mental illnesses. Children who lack sufficient human contact as they grow up develop serious psychological and physical problems that they even carry into their adult life.

Depression goes hand in hand with social isolation - being depressed makes you want shy away from social contact, which in turn makes you even feel more depressed. This vicious cycle is exacerbated when you feel unworthy of the company of others or you fear having to explain what you are going through.

However, if you suffer from depression, you must at all costs break out of that cycle and overcome this social isolation. It is impossible for your brain to function normally without social contact.

Human beings are by nature social creatures that need regular social contact to stay mentally healthy. Our brains and minds are shaped and function normally only when we are in continuous interaction with others.

The first place to look for improving your social contact is within your own inner circle; your loved ones and dear friends will almost always willingly offer their support if you muster the courage to open up to them.

Maintaining a certain level of social interaction in your life requires exerting a little bit of effort. You will have to reach out to others and often go outside your comfort zone. It is vital that you resist the urge to isolate yourself, as it will only lead you into a downwards spiral. Here are 4 tips to ensure you don't spend too much time by yourself:

Take up a new hobby

Very few things bring people together as naturally as common interests, so take advantage of that by joining a special interest group that caters to your preferred hobby (a knitting circle, a book or chess club...) This will not only help you maintain a healthy level of social contact, but it will occupy your mind and keep negative thoughts away.

Reconnect with old friends or family

If there is someone dear to you that you haven't spoken to in a while, pick up the phone or write them an email. You may feel reluctant to do this, but you'll be surprised how much better you feel after such a conversation.

Volunteer

Find a worthy cause in your neighborhood, such as homeless shelter and offer to help when you can. The experience of helping out others who are less fortunate than you can be enlightening. You will come out of it with a renewed appreciation for your own life and for the capacity of the human spirit to endure just about anything.

Open up to someone

Whether it's an old and trusted friend or a qualified therapist, you need to get talking about your condition and how you are moving along. You don't have to discuss everything at length right away but broaching the subject in a safe and non-judgmental environment will feel a like a weight off your shoulders.

Step 8 - Sunlight Exposure

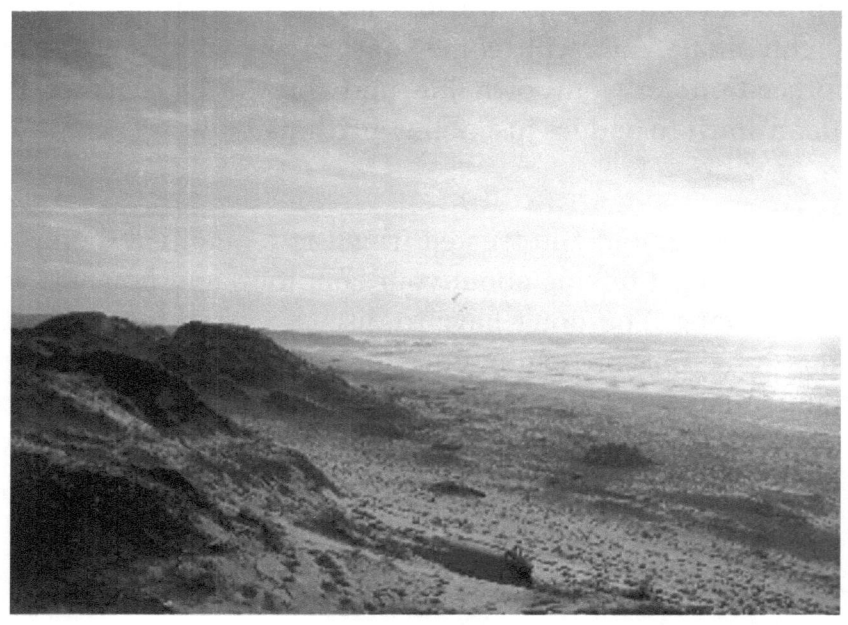

"When the sun is shining I can do anything; no mountain is too high, no trouble too difficult to overcome."
Wilma Rudolph

Millions of people around the world experience a form of depression every year during the dark months of winter when the sun disappears. This condition is called *seasonal affective disorder* and it originates from reduced exposure to sunlight during the cold and cloudy days of winter.

If you suffer from depression, one of the easiest ways to improve your mood is to go out in the sun. In the same way the sun banishes darkness when it rises, exposure to sunlight can significantly brighten up your mood.

The light that emanates from the sun replenishes your body's store of vitamin D (which plays an important role in mental health) and stimulates your body's production of serotonin – a neurotransmitter that regulates mood, appetite, sleep, and memory.

Exposure to sunlight adjusts your body clock for optimal function and regulates the circadian rhythms that dictate when you eat and fall asleep. It also improves irregular sleeping patterns like insomnia or hypersomnia. If you live in an area where sunlight is scarce, you can purchase sun lamps that artificially simulate natural sunlight.

As with everything else, sunlight should be enjoyed in moderation. Overexposure to the sun is detrimental to your health, so make sure to observe the following precautions before going out in the sun:

- **Pick the right time**: Early morning sunlight is best for your mood and for your health. It is therefore best to face the sun between 7 and 10 am. The intensity of sunlight during this time is more of gentle warmth rather than searing heat, as it tends to be subsequent hours of the day.

- **Put on sunscreen**: You want to enjoy the benefits of sunlight without suffering consequences like sunburn. If your skin normally burns after 10 minutes in the sun, applying sunscreen with an spf (sunburn protection factor) of 15 will allow you to stay under the sun for approximately two hours without sunburn.

- **Keep yourself hydrated**: Have a bottle of water next to you as you bask in the sun. Exposure to the sun speeds up your body's dehydration process, so you should take take regular sips of water to guard against this.

Step 9 - Quality Sleep

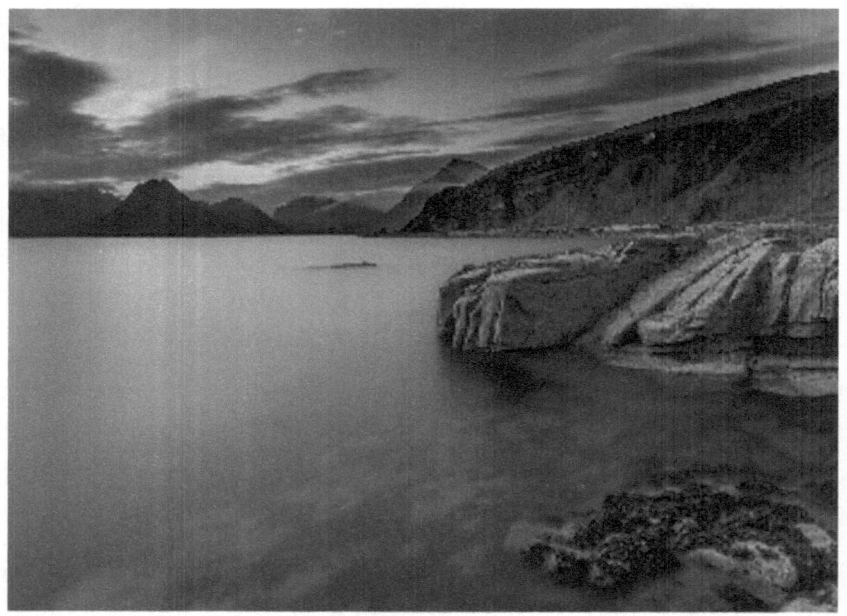

"If you can't sleep, then get up and do something instead of lying there worrying. It's the worry that gets you, not the lack of sleep."
Dale Carnegie

There is a definite but intricate relationship between sleep and depression: not only does depression cause sleep problems but sleep problems also cause depression. Sadly, the vast majority of depressed people are hostage to this vicious cycle of depression and lack of sleep.

Quality of sleep and mood are intrinsically linked. Only one night of poor sleep can significantly affect your mood the next day and even hinder your ability to think effectively. This is why prolonged episodes of sleep deprivation are one of the most potent triggers of depression.

Getting quality sleep every night is essential when it comes to overcoming depression. Simply put, quality sleep occurs when you are able to get uninterrupted sleep for about 6 to 8 hours, thus feeling rested upon waking up. Here are 5 ways you can achieve higher quality sleep:

Use your bedroom for sleep only

Re-establish your bedroom as a place reserved for sleeping. Once you are able to rid other associations (like work and entertainment) with your bedroom, sleep will come to you more naturally.

Power down

It's important to dim the lights, turn off the TVs, computers and other blue-light sources at least an hour before you go to bed. Blue light disrupts your slumber by suppressing melatonin, the hormone that brings about sleep.

Calm Your Mind

Meditate or pray before going to bed. One of the most potent factors that prevent you from falling asleep is a troubled mind. Meditation or prayer will clear your mind and help you fall asleep much quicker.

Establish a bedtime routine

Train your body to stick to a sleep schedule, even on weekends. Try to go to bed at the same time every night and wake up at the same time every morning, even when you don't have to. Having a consistent sleep routine keeps your internal clock in sync, which inevitably leads to better sleep.

Journal

If your worries are keeping you up at night, take a journal and start jotting down your concerns. You can even come up with an action plan to address each one. You'll be surprised how therapeutic this can be as it helps you get your worries out of your mind and on paper instead.

Step 10 - Practice Gratitude

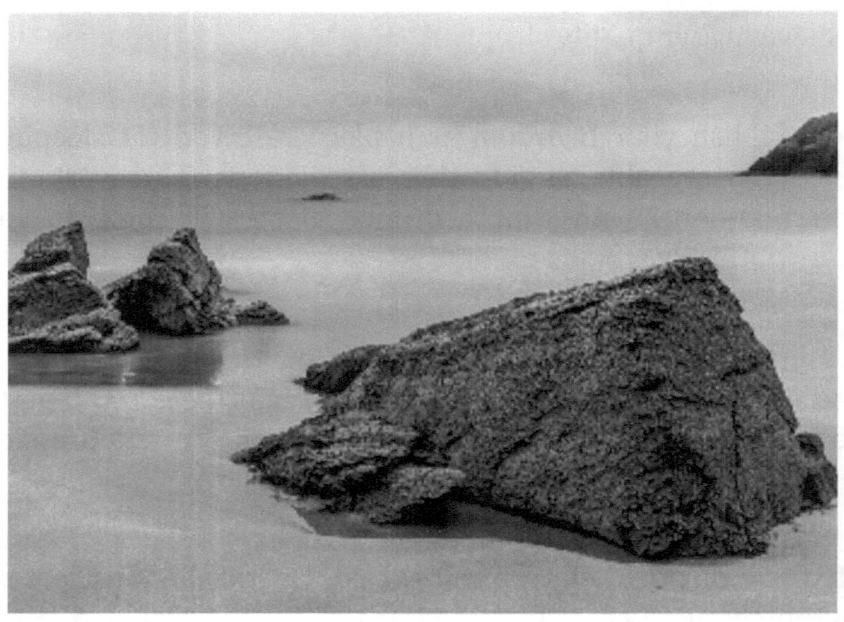

"Be thankful for what you have; you'll end up having more. If you concentrate on what you don't have, you will never, ever have enough."
Oprah Winfrey

The quality of your thinking reflects the quality of your life. Your dominant thoughts are what create your reality. In order to overcome depression, you must plant positive seeds in your mind by consistently replacing negative thoughts with more positive, empowering ones.

The most powerful way to start rewiring your brain for positivity is to start practicing gratitude. Consciously choosing to think of what you are grateful for is one of the most effective ways to reprogram your thought patterns.

Gilbert K. Chesterton says, "I would maintain that thanks are the highest form of thought, and that gratitude is happiness doubled by wonder."

In life, whatever you focus on expands. Focusing on positive thoughts and being grateful for the little things in your life will bring about even more good into your life and will have a tremendous impact on your mental wellbeing.

Everyone's life is comprised of positive and negative aspects, but all it takes to increase the quality of your life is to focus on all the things that you can be grateful for.

Here are some ways to practice gratitude in your daily life:

Focus on the Positive in You

Think about what you like about yourself. Depression can make anyone feel worthless and inferior, so to battle that, you need to focus on what makes you special. It can be as small as how your eyes light up when you smile or as profound as how well you take care of your children.

Keep a Gratitude Journal

Keep a gratitude journal and make it a habit to write down at least five things that you are thankful for every day. Ideally, this should be done before going to sleep as a calming exercise. You could be thankful for a healthy meal you enjoyed, your ability to see and hear, or the fact that you still have all your limbs functioning properly. Doing this everyday will transform your life.

Be Lavish in Your Praise

Aim to give out at least one compliment every day. It can be something as basic as telling a friend or a colleague that you like their scarf or their hairstyle. Mark Twain said, "I can live two months on a good compliment" Giving genuine compliments are one of the most powerful ways to strengthen your bonds with other people.

Stop complaining

Challenge yourself to keep from complaining, criticizing or gossiping about anything or anyone for the next 10 days. If you slip up, simply pull yourself back together and try again. You'll be surprised how much time energy you spent on negative thoughts.

Reframe Negative Thoughts

Train your mind to look for the positive in every situation. If you come across someone or something with a negative trait, find something positive about it. For instance, if you run into some heavy traffic on the way to work, focus on how you can use this time to listen to an audiobook or even meditate as you wait in traffic. Training your mind to reframe negative thoughts will improve the quality of your life.

Step 11 - Recondition Your Subconscious Mind

"The reason man may become the master of his own destiny is because he has the power to influence his own subconscious mind."
Napoleon Hill

I've always been passionate about the inner workings of the mind and recently I have created a resource that can help you reprogram your subconscious mind using subliminal messages.

If you've never heard of subliminal messages, they are simply visual or auditory stimuli that lie below the level of your conscious awareness.

Because you cannot consciously perceive them, subliminal messages go directly to your subconscious mind - the most powerful part of your mind that dictates 95% of your day-to-day thoughts and behaviors.

Back in March 2015, I created a YouTube Channel called Black Sheep (*type in "black sheep subliminal" on YouTube to find it*), where I offer high quality subliminal sessions to help people recondition their subconscious minds and thus their entire lives. The channel covers various topics such as wealth, health, relationships, self-confidence... I have recently created a session specifically to overcome depression and anxiety. You can use this session between one and six times a day to reprogram your subconscious mind to overcome depression.

Your subconscious mind is the driving force behind 95% of your day-to-day actions and behaviors. By reprogramming it you can effectively change your entire life and manifest anything you want.

Conclusion

I hope this book was able to help you to acquire a better understanding of depression and how you can take practical steps to overcome it without having to resort to prescription drugs and endure any dangerous side effects.

The next step is to consistently apply the techniques that you have learned in this book, keep learning about depression and keep making progress every single day. As Charlie Munger says, "Step by step you get ahead, but not necessarily in fast spurs. But you build discipline by preparing for fast spurts."

I wish you success on your path to recovery and I hope that reading this book has made you see a little bit of light at the end of the tunnel.

Finally, if you enjoyed this book, then I'd like to ask you a favor. Would you be kind enough to share your thoughts and post a review of this book on Amazon?

Your voice is important for this book to reach as many people as possible. The more reviews this book gets, the more people will be able to find it and become better equipped to overcome depression.

Thank you for getting this book and good luck on your journey towards a happier and healthier life!

Bonus: Free Guided Meditation Series (5 Audiobooks)

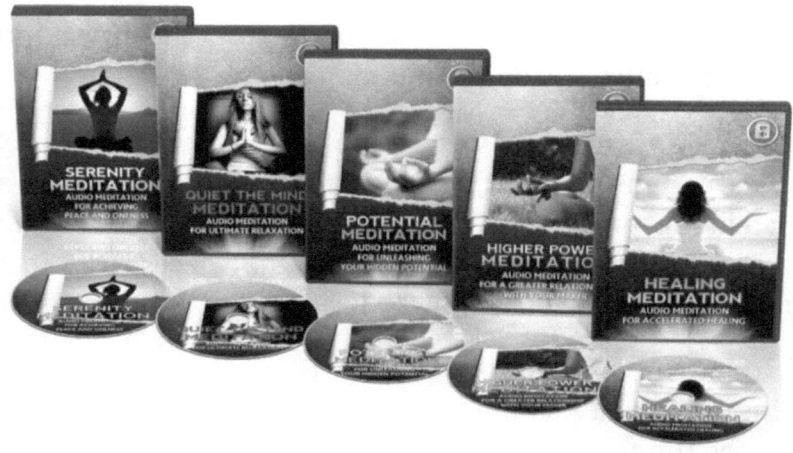

→ Go to www.projectlimitlesslife.com/bonus-2 to get your FREE Guided Meditation Series

You will get immediate access to:

- Healing Audio Meditation
- Higher Power Audio Meditation
- Potential Audio Meditation
- Quiet the Mind Audio Meditation
- Serenity Audio Meditation

You will also join my private kindle club and be the first to know about my upcoming books!

Preview of The Meditation Beginner's Bible

Get *The Meditation Beginner's Bible* at
http://amzn.to/1MR7wlu

Chapter 1 - What is meditation?

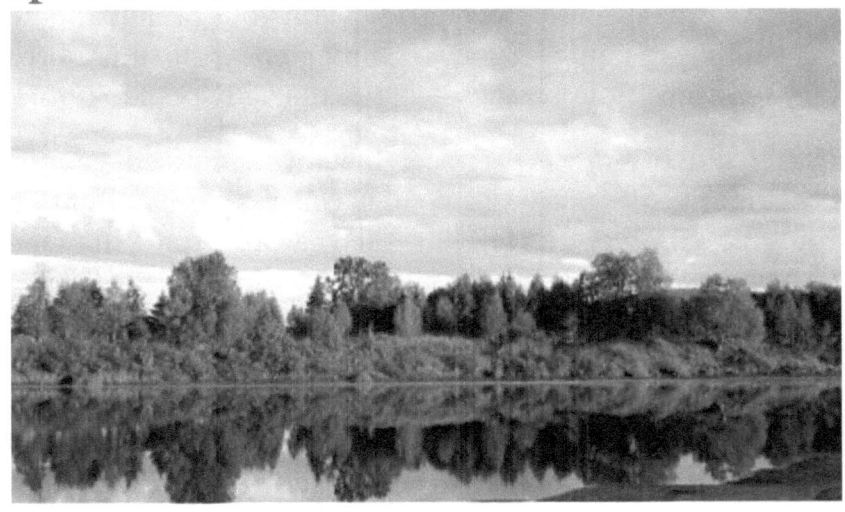

"The gift of learning to meditate is the greatest gift you can give yourself in this lifetime."
Sogyal Rinpoche

The word meditation and the word medicine come from the same Latin root "medicus" which means to cure. In the same way medicine cures sickness that exists inside the physical body by restoring it to a healthy state, meditation cures sickness that exists within the mind by returning it to its natural state of peace, joy and happiness.

But how does the mind become sick? Well, in our modern society most of us suffer from what we call compulsive thinking. We have this inner voice that is constantly thinking, ruminating the past, worrying about the future, and hence we never fully experience the present moment.

Take a few seconds right now and become aware of your breathing. Observe the changing sensations of your breath as you inhale and then exhale. Be aware of your lungs filling and emptying themselves. Become one with your breath and notice the subtle gap between your incoming and outcoming breath - let yourself completely dissolve into the activity of breathing.

If you did this little exercise, I bet you noticed your mind becoming a bit more still. When you rest your attention on your breath, you effectively step away from the chaotic impulses of the mind and you connect to your true Self – that eternal part of you that is beyond the ephemeral, ever-wavering physical realm.

Meditation is essentially a vehicle for accessing a higher level of consciousness that is beyond thought, where you are reconnected to your deepest self, your true nature of joy, peace and happiness. When you meditate, you effectively increase your level of self-awareness and you awaken to the things that are beyond thought - love, beauty, peace... This cannot be rationalized intellectually; however it can be experienced when you bring stillness into your mind.

Moreover, meditation does not require effort. As mentioned earlier, it is not about trying to empty your mind. Spiritual leader Deepak Chopra puts it beautifully: "*Meditation is not a way of making your mind quiet. It is a way of entering into the quiet that is already there - buried under the 50 000 thoughts the average person thinks everyday.*"

When you practice meditation, you gain control over your mind, you break the cycle of seeking stimulation from the external world and you learn to draw your state from within. Meditation is truly a transformative experience that can have profound effects not just on your mind, but on virtually every aspect of your life – your body, relationships, health and even your career.

Chapter 2 - The Benefits of Meditation

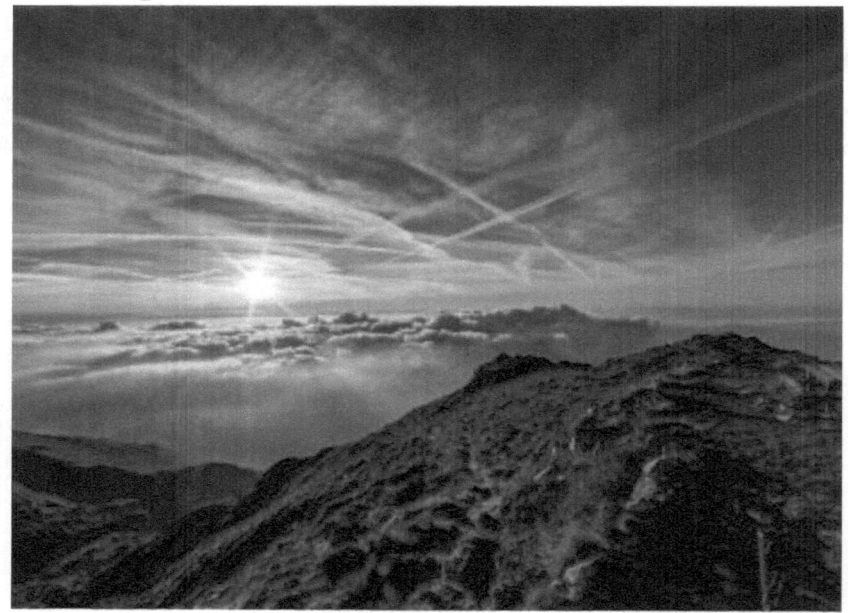

"Meditation more than anything in my life was the biggest ingredient of whatever success I've had."
Ray Dalio

Over the past decade, a vast amount of scientific research has been carried out to investigate the benefits of meditation for the human mind and body. The National Institute of Health has spent over $100 million toward research on meditation, and nowadays it seems like new studies professing the benefits of meditation are emerging everyday.

As a result of the various scientific discoveries on the benefits of meditation, a growing number of hospitals and medical centers are now teaching meditation to patients in order to address various health ailments, relieve pain and fight stress. For example, one famous meditation program called *Mindfulness Based Stress Reduction*, which was created in

1979 by Dr Jon Kabat-Zinn has become so popular that it is now offered in over 200 medical centers around the world.

One remarkable example of the effectiveness of meditation for pain relief is shown in a study conducted by Dr Fadel Zeidan at the Wake Forest Medical Center in North Carolina. In the study, 15 people who had never practiced meditation attended four, 20-minute mindfulness meditation classes. The participants' brain activity was examined before and after the training using magnetic resonance imaging. During both scans, they were exposed to a pain-inducing heat device. The results were impressive: After the training, the participant's pain intensity was reduced by about 40% and their pain unpleasantness by around 57%: 80 minutes of meditation was more effective than pain relieving drugs like morphine, which normally reduces pain by about 25%.

Meditation has also become popular in the corporate world, with some leading companies like Google providing meditation classes to their employees to relieve stress, improve focus and boost productivity. The search giant even took it a step further by building a labyrinth to encourage the practice of walking meditation. Moreover, Google is not the only company that is embracing meditation. In fact, other big corporations like Apple, Nike, Yahoo, McKinsey & Co... have all brought meditation to their workplaces in an endeavor to keep employees happy and productive.

Even schools are now adopting meditation to make kids calmer and more focused. Youth meditation program are being installed everywhere in the US, England, Canada and India. In 2014, Educational Psychology Review examined 15 peer-reviewed studies on meditation in schools and concluded that the practice had a myriad of positive effects on students, such as lessened anxiety, increased focus and stronger friendships.

Over 3,000 scientific studies have now been conducted on the benefits of meditation and the truth is practicing meditation has so many benefits that I could not list them all in this book. So here are 53 noteworthy benefits of developing a regular meditation practice:

Health Benefits

- Lowers blood pressure more effectively than medication
- Relieves pain more effectively than morphine
- Slows the progression of HIV
- Helps prevent fibromyalgia and arthritis
- Reduces risk of Alzheimer's
- Reduces risk of heart disease and stroke
- Provides rest deeper than sleep
- Helps recover from addiction
- Improves cardiovascular function
- Relieves irritable bowel syndrome
- Increases energy levels
- Slows down the aging process
- Improves athletic performance
- Improves quality of sleep
- Improves fertility
- Decreases muscle tension
- Improves skin tone
- Increases air flow to the lungs
- Boosts the immune system
- Reduces inflammation

Mental and Emotional Benefits

- Improves attention, focus and ability to work under pressure
- Helps manage ADHD
- Improves intelligence and memory
- Improves critical thinking and decision-making
- Fosters creativity
- Slows down cognitive decline
- Builds composure and calm in all situations
- Increases brain connectivity
- Improves mental strength
- Improves sex life
- Cultivates willpower
- Boosts cognitive function
- Increases grey matter in the hippocampus and frontal areas of the brain
- Helps manage emotional eating
- Promotes good mood
- Improves working memory and executive functioning
- Helps beat depression
- Reduces stress and anxiety
- Improves emotional stability
- Fosters empathy and positive relationships
- Decreases feelings of nervousness
- Reduces social isolation
- Enhances feelings of happiness and vitality
- Improves communication with other people
- Develops a sense of calm and serenity

Spiritual Benefits

- Enhances self-awareness
- Fosters peace of mind, happiness and joy
- Increases self-acceptance
- Boosts self-compassion
- Increases self-esteem
- Develops intuition
- Builds wisdom
- Increases capacity for love

→ *Get The Meditation Beginner's Bible* at
http://amzn.to/1MR7wlu